DR. BARBARA'S GUIDE TO REVERSING AND HEALING DIABETES

Unlocking wellness: Dr. Barbara's proven strategies for reversing diabetes. Transform your health with expert guidance and holistic healing method

I0781592

Odesa mulan

Table of Contents

COPYRIGHT © 2023

CHAPTER ONE

Introduction to Dr. Barbara's Approach to Reversing Diabetes

In recent years, the prevalence of diabetes has surged globally, becoming one of the most pressing health concerns of the 21st century. With approximately 463 million adults living with diabetes worldwide in 2019, according to the International Diabetes Federation (IDF), the urgency to find effective treatments and prevention strategies has never been greater. Amidst this health crisis, Dr. Barbara's approach to reversing diabetes has garnered attention for its holistic and comprehensive methodology.

Dr. Barbara, a renowned endocrinologist and researcher, has dedicated her career to unraveling the complexities of diabetes and developing innovative approaches to combat this disease. Her methodology emphasizes not only managing symptoms but also addressing the root causes of diabetes to achieve lasting reversal and improved overall health. By integrating elements of nutrition, exercise, stress management, and personalized medical interventions, Dr. Barbara's approach offers hope to millions of individuals grappling with diabetes.

Understanding Diabetes: A Brief Overview

Before delving into Dr. Barbara's approach, it is crucial to understand the fundamental mechanisms of diabetes. Diabetes mellitus is a chronic metabolic disorder characterized by elevated blood glucose levels, resulting from either insufficient insulin production, ineffective insulin utilization, or both. Insulin, produced by the pancreas, plays a central role in regulating blood sugar levels by facilitating the uptake of glucose into cells for energy production.

Type 1 diabetes, often diagnosed in childhood or adolescence, is an autoimmune condition where the immune system attacks and destroys insulin-producing beta cells in the pancreas, leading to an absolute insulin deficiency. On the other hand, type 2 diabetes, the most common form, typically develops in adulthood and is closely linked to lifestyle factors such as obesity, sedentary behavior, and poor dietary choices. In type 2 diabetes, cells become resistant to the effects of insulin, causing glucose to accumulate in the bloodstream.

Challenges in Diabetes Management

Conventional approaches to diabetes management primarily focus on symptom control through medication, insulin therapy, and lifestyle modifications. While these interventions are essential for glycemic control and preventing complications, they often fall short in achieving sustained reversal of the disease.

Moreover, the increasing prevalence of diabetes and its associated economic burden underscore the need for more effective and scalable solutions.

One of the major challenges in diabetes management is the reliance on pharmacotherapy, which may lead to side effects, treatment fatigue, and financial strain on healthcare systems and individuals. Additionally, lifestyle interventions, such as diet and exercise, are often difficult to maintain long-term, contributing to the relapse of diabetes symptoms. Furthermore, the heterogeneity of diabetes presentations and individual responses to treatment necessitate personalized approaches tailored to each patient's unique needs.

Dr. Barbara's Holistic Approach

Dr. Barbara's approach to reversing diabetes embodies a holistic and patient-centered philosophy that goes beyond traditional disease management strategies. At the core of her methodology is the recognition that diabetes is a multifactorial condition influenced by genetic predisposition, environmental factors, and lifestyle choices. By addressing the interconnectedness of these factors, Dr. Barbara aims to restore metabolic health and reverse the underlying drivers of diabetes.

Central to Dr. Barbara's approach is the emphasis on nutrition as a cornerstone of diabetes reversal. She advocates for a whole-food, plant-based diet rich in fruits, vegetables, legumes, and whole grains, while minimizing processed foods, refined sugars, and saturated fats. This dietary pattern not only helps stabilize blood sugar levels but also promotes weight loss, improves insulin sensitivity, and reduces inflammation, all of which are critical for reversing diabetes.

In addition to dietary modifications, Dr. Barbara emphasizes the importance of regular physical activity in diabetes reversal. Exercise helps lower blood glucose levels, improve insulin sensitivity, and support weight management. Moreover, physical activity has numerous cardiovascular and psychological benefits, further enhancing overall health and well-being in individuals with diabetes.

Personalized Medicine and Precision Health

Another key aspect of Dr. Barbara's approach is personalized medicine, which involves tailoring treatment strategies to each patient's unique biological characteristics, genetic makeup, lifestyle factors, and preferences. By leveraging advances in genomics, metabolomics, and digital health technologies, Dr. Barbara aims to identify biomarkers and predictive markers that can guide personalized interventions and optimize outcomes in diabetes reversal.

Through comprehensive medical assessments and diagnostic tests, Dr. Barbara evaluates various metabolic parameters, including insulin sensitivity, beta-cell function, lipid profiles, and inflammatory markers. Armed with this data, she develops personalized treatment plans that may include targeted medications, supplements, and lifestyle modifications tailored to each individual's specific needs and goals.

Furthermore, Dr. Barbara recognizes the importance of addressing psychosocial factors in diabetes management, such as stress, depression, and social support. Chronic stress and mental health issues can adversely affect glycemic control and exacerbate diabetes complications. Therefore, Dr. Barbara incorporates stress management techniques, mindfulness practices, and behavioral therapy into her treatment approach to promote emotional well-being and resilience in her patients.

Evidence-Based Practices and Research Initiatives

Dr. Barbara's approach to reversing diabetes is grounded in scientific evidence and informed by ongoing research initiatives aimed at advancing our understanding of the disease and optimizing treatment strategies. She actively collaborates with interdisciplinary teams of researchers, clinicians, and industry partners to conduct clinical trials, observational studies, and translational research projects focused on diabetes prevention, reversal, and management.

Through rigorous scientific inquiry and data-driven decision-making, Dr. Barbara seeks to identify novel therapeutic targets, biomarkers, and interventions that can enhance the efficacy and sustainability of diabetes reversal efforts. Moreover, she is committed to disseminating research findings through peer-reviewed publications, conferences, and public outreach initiatives to inform healthcare providers, policymakers, and the general public about the latest advancements in diabetes care.

Conclusion

In conclusion, Dr. Barbara's approach to reversing diabetes offers a comprehensive and personalized framework for addressing the complex interplay of genetic, environmental, and lifestyle factors underlying this prevalent metabolic disorder. By integrating nutrition, exercise, personalized medicine, and psychosocial support, Dr. Barbara aims to empower individuals with diabetes to take control of their health and achieve sustainable reversal of the disease. Through evidence-based practices, research initiatives, and a patient-centered philosophy, Dr. Barbara continues to pave the way for innovative solutions in diabetes care, bringing hope to millions of individuals worldwide affected by this chronic condition.

CHAPTER TWO

Understanding Diabetes: Types, Symptoms, and Complications

Diabetes is a chronic metabolic disorder characterized by elevated blood sugar levels, resulting from either insufficient insulin production, ineffective insulin utilization, or both. This condition affects millions of people worldwide and can lead to serious health complications if left unmanaged. Understanding the different types of diabetes, their symptoms, and potential complications is crucial for effective management and prevention strategies.

Types of Diabetes

1. **Type 1 Diabetes (T1D)**:

   - Type 1 diabetes, also known as insulin-dependent diabetes or juvenile diabetes, typically develops in childhood or adolescence but can occur at any age.

   - It is an autoimmune condition where the immune system mistakenly attacks and destroys insulin-producing beta cells in the pancreas.

   - As a result, individuals with type 1 diabetes have an absolute deficiency of insulin and require lifelong insulin therapy for survival.

- The exact cause of type 1 diabetes is not fully understood, but genetic predisposition and environmental factors, such as viral infections, may play a role.

2. **Type 2 Diabetes (T2D)**:

- Type 2 diabetes is the most common form of diabetes, accounting for the majority of cases worldwide.

- It typically develops in adulthood, although there has been a concerning rise in its prevalence among children and adolescents due to increasing rates of obesity and sedentary lifestyles.

- In type 2 diabetes, cells become resistant to the effects of insulin, and the pancreas may fail to produce enough insulin to overcome this resistance.

- Risk factors for type 2 diabetes include obesity, physical inactivity, unhealthy diet, family history of diabetes, and ethnicity.

3. **Gestational Diabetes Mellitus (GDM)**:

- Gestational diabetes mellitus occurs during pregnancy and is characterized by high blood sugar levels that develop or are first recognized during pregnancy.

- Hormonal changes, increased insulin resistance, and genetic factors contribute to the development of gestational diabetes.

- Although gestational diabetes usually resolves after childbirth, women who have had gestational diabetes are at increased risk of developing type 2 diabetes later in life.

4. **Other Types of Diabetes**:

- Other less common types of diabetes include monogenic diabetes, which is caused by mutations in a single gene, and secondary diabetes, which results from underlying medical conditions such as pancreatitis, hormonal disorders, or medication use.

Symptoms of Diabetes

The symptoms of diabetes can vary depending on the type of diabetes and the individual's metabolic status. However, common symptoms of diabetes include:

1. **Polyuria (Frequent Urination)**: Excess glucose in the bloodstream leads to increased urine production, causing frequent urination.

2. **Polydipsia (Excessive Thirst)**: Dehydration resulting from frequent urination triggers excessive thirst.

3. **Polyphagia (Increased Hunger)**: Inadequate insulin action prevents glucose from entering cells for energy, leading to increased hunger.

4. **Unexplained Weight Loss**: Despite increased hunger and food intake, individuals with diabetes may experience unexplained weight loss due to the body's inability to utilize glucose effectively.

5. **Fatigue**: Insufficient glucose uptake by cells results in reduced energy production, leading to fatigue and weakness.

6. **Blurred Vision**: High blood sugar levels can cause changes in the shape of the lens in the eye, leading to blurred vision.

7. **Slow Healing of Wounds**: Diabetes impairs the body's ability to repair damaged tissues and wounds, resulting in slow wound healing.

8. **Recurrent Infections**: High blood sugar levels weaken the immune system, making individuals with diabetes more susceptible to infections, such as urinary tract infections, skin infections, and yeast infections.

It is important to note that some individuals with type 2 diabetes may not experience noticeable symptoms initially, and the condition may be diagnosed during routine blood tests or screening.

Complications of Diabetes

Untreated or poorly managed diabetes can lead to a range of acute and chronic complications affecting various organ systems in the body. Some of the common complications of diabetes include:

1. **Cardiovascular Disease**: Diabetes significantly increases the risk of developing cardiovascular diseases such as coronary artery disease, heart attack, stroke, and peripheral arterial disease.

2. **Nephropathy (Kidney Disease)**: Diabetes is a leading cause of kidney failure, characterized by progressive damage to the kidneys' filtering units (glomeruli) and impaired kidney function.

3. **Neuropathy (Nerve Damage)**: Elevated blood sugar levels can damage nerves throughout the body, leading to peripheral neuropathy, which causes numbness, tingling, pain, and weakness, particularly in the hands and feet.

4. **Retinopathy (Eye Damage)**: Diabetes can cause damage to the blood vessels in the retina, leading to diabetic retinopathy, a leading cause of blindness in adults.

5. **Foot Complications**: Nerve damage and poor blood circulation in the feet increase the risk of foot ulcers, infections, and, in severe cases, lower limb amputations.

6. **Skin Complications**: Diabetes increases the risk of various skin conditions, including bacterial and fungal infections, diabetic dermopathy, and necrobiosis lipoidicadiabeticorum.

7. **Hypoglycemia (Low Blood Sugar)**: Intensive insulin therapy or certain diabetes medications can cause blood sugar levels to drop too low, resulting in hypoglycemia, which can lead to confusion, seizures, and loss of consciousness if left untreated.

These complications underscore the importance of early diagnosis, optimal glycemic control, and comprehensive diabetes management to prevent or delay the progression of diabetes-related complications and improve overall quality of life for individuals living with diabetes.

In summary, diabetes is a complex metabolic disorder characterized by elevated blood sugar levels and impaired insulin function. Understanding the different types of diabetes, recognizing common symptoms, and being aware of potential complications are essential for early diagnosis, effective management, and prevention strategies. With proper medical care, lifestyle modifications, and adherence to treatment regimens, individuals with diabetes can lead fulfilling lives and reduce their risk of long-term complications.

CHAPTER THREE

The Philosophy Behind Dr. Barbara's Herbal Approach

Dr. Barbara's herbal approach to health and wellness is grounded in the principles of holistic medicine, which views the body as a complex interconnected system that strives for balance and optimal functioning. Central to her philosophy is the belief in the innate healing power of nature and the importance of addressing the underlying root causes of illness rather than merely treating symptoms. Dr. Barbara's herbal approach draws upon traditional wisdom, scientific research, and clinical expertise to harness the therapeutic properties of herbs and botanical remedies in promoting health, vitality, and longevity.

Holistic Healing and Wellness

At the heart of Dr. Barbara's herbal approach is the recognition that true healing encompasses the physical, mental, emotional, and spiritual dimensions of an individual. She views health not merely as the absence of disease but as a state of harmony and equilibrium within the body, mind, and spirit. By adopting a holistic perspective, Dr. Barbara seeks to identify and address the underlying imbalances or disruptions that contribute to illness and restore the body's natural ability to heal itself.

Natural Remedies and Botanical Medicine

Herbal medicine, also known as botanical medicine or phytotherapy, forms the cornerstone of Dr. Barbara's approach to health and wellness. She believes that plants contain a myriad of bioactive compounds with powerful healing properties that have been utilized by diverse cultures for centuries. From ancient Ayurvedic traditions to indigenous healing practices, the therapeutic potential of herbs has been revered and passed down through generations.

Dr. Barbara harnesses the wisdom of traditional herbalism and combines it with modern scientific research to develop evidence-based herbal formulations and treatment protocols tailored to individual needs. She selects herbs based on their specific actions, synergistic effects, and safety profiles, taking into account factors such as dosage, potency, and method of administration to optimize therapeutic outcomes.

Principles of Herbalism

Dr. Barbara's herbal approach is guided by several key principles of herbalism:

1. **Individualization**: Recognizing that each person is unique, Dr. Barbara emphasizes the importance of personalized herbal protocols tailored to an individual's constitution, health status, and therapeutic goals.

2. **Whole-Plant Medicine**: Rather than isolating single compounds, Dr. Barbara prefers to utilize whole-plant extracts or herbal preparations that preserve the full spectrum of bioactive constituents, synergistic interactions, and inherent healing properties of the plant.

3. **Safety and Quality**: Ensuring the safety and quality of herbal remedies is paramount. Dr. Barbara sources herbs from reputable suppliers, adheres to Good Manufacturing Practices (GMP), and conducts rigorous quality control measures to ensure purity, potency, and consistency.

4. **Education and Empowerment**: Dr. Barbara believes in empowering individuals to take an active role in their health and well-being. She provides education, guidance, and support to help clients make informed decisions about herbal remedies, lifestyle modifications, and self-care practices.

5. **Integration with Conventional Medicine**: While herbal medicine is central to her approach, Dr. Barbara recognizes the value of integrating complementary therapies with conventional medical treatments when appropriate. She collaborates with healthcare providers to ensure safe and effective integration of herbal remedies into comprehensive treatment plans.

Promoting Balance and Vitality

The overarching goal of Dr. Barbara's herbal approach is to promote balance, vitality, and resilience within the body. Whether addressing acute health concerns or chronic conditions, her focus is on restoring harmony to the body's systems, enhancing immune function, supporting detoxification pathways, and nourishing vital organs and tissues.

By embracing the philosophy of holistic healing, harnessing the healing power of plants, and empowering individuals to take charge of their health, Dr. Barbara's herbal approach offers a natural and integrative path to wellness that honors the body's innate wisdom and capacity for healing.

CHAPTER FOUR

Preparing for Treatment: Mental and Physical Readiness

Preparing for medical treatment, whether it's surgery, chemotherapy, or any other intervention, involves more than just physical readiness. Mental and emotional preparedness are equally important aspects that can significantly influence the outcome and experience of the treatment process. Dr. Barbara emphasizes the holistic approach to preparing for treatment, focusing on both mental and physical aspects to optimize the overall well-being of the individual undergoing medical care.

Mental Readiness

1. **Understanding the Procedure**: One of the first steps in mental readiness is to gain a clear understanding of the treatment procedure, including its purpose, potential risks and benefits, and expected outcomes. This knowledge helps alleviate anxiety and uncertainty, empowering individuals to make informed decisions about their care.

2. **Managing Expectations**: It's essential to have realistic expectations about the treatment process and its outcomes. While medical interventions aim to improve health and quality of life, they may not always yield immediate or perfect results. Dr. Barbara encourages open communication

with healthcare providers to address any concerns or questions and establish realistic goals for treatment.

3. **Coping Strategies**: Coping with the stress and emotional challenges of undergoing medical treatment requires effective coping strategies. These may include mindfulness techniques, relaxation exercises, deep breathing, visualization, or seeking support from friends, family, or mental health professionals. Dr. Barbara emphasizes the importance of finding coping strategies that resonate with the individual's preferences and personality.

4. **Building Resilience**: Cultivating resilience is key to navigating the ups and downs of the treatment journey. Resilience involves adapting to adversity, maintaining a positive outlook, and drawing upon inner strength and resources to overcome challenges. Dr. Barbara encourages individuals to tap into their resilience by focusing on their strengths, nurturing supportive relationships, and fostering a sense of purpose and meaning in life.

5. **Addressing Emotional Needs**: It's normal to experience a range of emotions, including fear, anxiety, sadness, or anger, when facing medical treatment. Dr. Barbara emphasizes the importance of acknowledging and expressing these emotions in a healthy and constructive manner. Seeking professional counseling or participating in support groups can provide a

safe space to process emotions and gain perspective from others who have faced similar challenges.

Physical Readiness

1. **Optimizing Physical Health**: Prior to undergoing treatment, it's essential to optimize physical health to enhance the body's ability to tolerate and recover from medical interventions. This may involve following a balanced diet, engaging in regular exercise, getting adequate sleep, and managing chronic health conditions such as diabetes, hypertension, or obesity.

2. **Medication Management**: If the treatment involves medications, it's important to review and manage current medications in consultation with healthcare providers. This includes ensuring proper dosages, understanding potential drug interactions, and adhering to prescribed regimens.

3. **Preoperative Preparation**: For surgical procedures, preoperative preparation may include fasting instructions, bowel preparation, cessation of certain medications (such as blood thinners), and preoperative tests or evaluations to assess overall health and identify any potential risks or contraindications.

4. **Rehabilitation Planning**: Depending on the type of treatment, rehabilitation planning may be necessary to facilitate recovery and restore function. This may involve

physical therapy, occupational therapy, speech therapy, or other rehabilitative interventions tailored to the individual's specific needs and goals.

5. **Social Support and Practical Assistance**: Having a strong support system in place can significantly aid in physical readiness for treatment. This may involve enlisting the help of family members, friends, or caregivers to assist with transportation, household chores, meal preparation, or childcare during the treatment process.

In summary, preparing for medical treatment involves comprehensive readiness, encompassing both mental and physical aspects. By fostering mental resilience, addressing emotional needs, optimizing physical health, and coordinating practical aspects of care, individuals can enhance their overall readiness for treatment and improve their ability to cope with the challenges and demands of the medical journey. Dr. Barbara's holistic approach emphasizes the importance of holistic well-being in preparing for treatment, recognizing that mental and physical health are interconnected and essential components of overall wellness.

CHAPTER FIVE

The Herbal Treatment Protocol: Overview and Guidelines

Dr. Barbara's herbal treatment protocol offers a holistic and personalized approach to promoting health and wellness using botanical remedies and natural interventions. Grounded in the principles of traditional herbalism and supported by scientific evidence, her protocol aims to address the root causes of health imbalances, restore vitality, and support the body's innate healing mechanisms. This overview provides a comprehensive guide to Dr. Barbara's herbal treatment protocol, outlining key principles, guidelines, and considerations for its implementation.

Principles of Herbal Treatment

1. **Holistic Approach**: Dr. Barbara's herbal treatment protocol adopts a holistic perspective, recognizing the interconnectedness of body, mind, and spirit in achieving optimal health. It addresses underlying imbalances and promotes wellness on multiple levels, encompassing physical, mental, emotional, and spiritual aspects of well-being.

2. **Individualization**: Herbal treatment plans are tailored to the unique needs, health status, and constitutional characteristics of each individual. Dr. Barbara considers

factors such as age, gender, medical history, lifestyle, dietary habits, and environmental influences to develop personalized protocols that optimize therapeutic outcomes.

3. **Whole-Plant Medicine**: Emphasizing the synergy of whole-plant extracts, Dr. Barbara utilizes herbal formulations that preserve the full spectrum of bioactive compounds and phytonutrients present in the plant. This approach enhances the therapeutic potency and therapeutic effects of herbal remedies compared to isolated compounds.

4. **Evidence-Based Practice**: Dr. Barbara's herbal treatment protocol is grounded in scientific research, clinical evidence, and traditional knowledge. She integrates the latest findings from botanical research with empirical observations and clinical experience to inform treatment decisions and optimize efficacy and safety.

5. **Safety and Quality Assurance**: Ensuring the safety and quality of herbal remedies is paramount. Dr. Barbara sources herbs from reputable suppliers, adheres to Good Manufacturing Practices (GMP), and conducts rigorous quality control measures to ensure purity, potency, and consistency.

Guidelines for Herbal Treatment

1. **Initial Assessment**: The herbal treatment process begins with a comprehensive assessment of the individual's health

history, current symptoms, lifestyle factors, and treatment goals. This assessment helps Dr. Barbara identify underlying imbalances, assess contraindications, and develop a personalized treatment plan.

2. **Herbal Formulations**: Based on the assessment findings, Dr. Barbara selects specific herbs and botanical remedies tailored to address the individual's unique needs and health concerns. Herbal formulations may include tinctures, teas, capsules, powders, or topical preparations, depending on the desired therapeutic effects and mode of administration.

3. **Dosage and Administration**: Herbal remedies are prescribed at appropriate dosages and frequencies to optimize therapeutic outcomes while minimizing the risk of adverse effects. Dosage recommendations take into account factors such as age, weight, sensitivity, and the severity of symptoms. Dr. Barbara provides clear instructions on how to administer herbal remedies safely and effectively.

4. **Monitoring and Adjustment**: Throughout the course of herbal treatment, Dr. Barbara monitors the individual's response to therapy, assesses progress, and makes any necessary adjustments to the treatment plan. This may involve modifying dosages, incorporating additional herbs, or discontinuing certain remedies based on changes in symptoms or health status.

5. **Lifestyle Modifications**: In addition to herbal remedies, Dr. Barbara emphasizes the importance of lifestyle modifications in promoting health and wellness. This may include dietary changes, stress management techniques, exercise routines, sleep hygiene practices, and environmental modifications tailored to support the individual's healing journey.

6. **Follow-Up and Support**: Regular follow-up appointments allow Dr. Barbara to track progress, address any concerns or questions, and provide ongoing support and guidance throughout the treatment process. Open communication and collaboration between the individual and Dr. Barbara are essential for optimizing therapeutic outcomes and promoting patient empowerment.

Considerations for Herbal Treatment

1. **Potential Interactions**: Herbal remedies may interact with medications, supplements, or underlying health conditions. It's important for individuals to disclose all medications, supplements, and health concerns to Dr. Barbara to minimize the risk of adverse interactions and ensure safe and effective treatment.

2. **Patient Education**: Educating individuals about herbal remedies, their therapeutic effects, and proper usage is essential for promoting adherence and empowering patients to take an active role in their health. Dr. Barbara provides

clear and comprehensive information about herbal treatments, including potential benefits, risks, and precautions.

3. **Long-Term Maintenance**: Herbal treatment is often integrated into a comprehensive wellness plan aimed at promoting long-term health and preventing future imbalances or health concerns. Dr. Barbara may recommend periodic maintenance doses or lifestyle modifications to sustain the benefits of herbal treatment and support ongoing well-being.

In summary, Dr. Barbara's herbal treatment protocol offers a holistic and individualized approach to promoting health and wellness using botanical remedies. By adhering to key principles, guidelines, and considerations outlined in this overview, individuals can experience the benefits of herbal treatment while minimizing risks and optimizing therapeutic outcomes. Collaboration between the individual and Dr. Barbara is essential for tailoring treatment plans to meet the unique needs and goals of each individual and supporting their journey toward optimal health and vitality.

CHAPTER SIX

Key Herbs and Plants Used in Dr. Barbara's Diabetes Reversal Plan

Dr. Barbara's diabetes reversal plan integrates a variety of herbs and plants known for their therapeutic properties in promoting metabolic health, improving insulin sensitivity, and supporting overall well-being. These botanical remedies are carefully selected based on their traditional uses, scientific evidence, and compatibility with individual needs and health goals. Here are some key herbs and plants commonly used in Dr. Barbara's diabetes reversal plan:

1. **Gymnema Sylvestre**:

   - Gymnemasylvestre is a perennial woody vine native to India and Africa, traditionally used in Ayurvedic medicine to support blood sugar control.

   - Studies suggest that gymnemasylvestre may help reduce blood sugar levels by blocking sugar absorption in the intestine, increasing insulin secretion, and improving insulin sensitivity.

   - Dr. Barbara may recommend gymnemasylvestre as part of a comprehensive diabetes reversal plan to help regulate blood glucose levels and support overall metabolic health.

2. **Cinnamon**:

- Cinnamon is a popular spice derived from the inner bark of several tree species belonging to the genus Cinnamomum.

- Research indicates that cinnamon may have antidiabetic effects, including improving insulin sensitivity, enhancing glucose uptake by cells, and reducing fasting blood sugar levels.

- Dr. Barbara may incorporate cinnamon into dietary recommendations or herbal formulations to help individuals with diabetes manage blood sugar levels and reduce insulin resistance.

3. **Bitter Melon**:

- Bitter melon, also known as bitter gourd or Momordica charantia, is a tropical vine widely cultivated for its edible fruit and medicinal properties.

- Bitter melon contains bioactive compounds, such as charantin, polypeptide-p, and vicine, which have been shown to exhibit hypoglycemic effects by improving insulin secretion and glucose utilization.

- Dr. Barbara may recommend bitter melon supplementation or include bitter melon extract in herbal formulations to help lower blood sugar levels and support diabetes management.

4. **Fenugreek**:

- Fenugreek, or Trigonella foenum-graecum, is an herbaceous plant native to the Mediterranean region and South Asia, valued for its culinary and medicinal uses.

- Studies suggest that fenugreek seeds and extracts may have antidiabetic properties, including improving glycemic control, reducing insulin resistance, and enhancing insulin secretion.

- Dr. Barbara may incorporate fenugreek into herbal formulations or dietary recommendations to help individuals with diabetes regulate blood glucose levels and improve metabolic parameters.

5. **Ginseng**:

- Ginseng is a perennial plant belonging to the Panax genus, prized in traditional Chinese medicine for its adaptogenic and tonic properties.

- Research suggests that ginseng may have beneficial effects on glucose metabolism, insulin sensitivity, and pancreatic function, making it potentially useful in diabetes management.

- Dr. Barbara may recommend ginseng supplementation or include ginseng extract in herbal formulations to support energy levels, reduce stress, and improve overall metabolic health in individuals with diabetes.

6. **Turmeric**:

- Turmeric, derived from the rhizomes of Curcuma longa, is a vibrant yellow spice commonly used in culinary and medicinal preparations.

- Curcumin, the main bioactive compound in turmeric, exhibits antioxidant, anti-inflammatory, and antidiabetic properties, which may help improve insulin sensitivity, reduce inflammation, and protect against diabetes-related complications.

- Dr. Barbara may recommend turmeric supplementation or include turmeric extract in herbal formulations to support immune function, reduce oxidative stress, and mitigate inflammation in individuals with diabetes.

7. **Ginger**:

- Ginger, derived from the rhizome of Zingiber officinale, is a versatile herb with a long history of medicinal use in traditional healing systems.

- Ginger contains bioactive compounds, such as gingerol and shogaol, which possess antioxidant, anti-inflammatory, and antidiabetic properties, potentially beneficial for individuals with diabetes.

- Dr. Barbara may incorporate ginger into dietary recommendations, herbal formulations, or teas to help manage blood sugar levels, improve digestion, and reduce inflammation in individuals with diabetes.

These key herbs and plants are just a few examples of the diverse botanical remedies that Dr. Barbara may include in her diabetes reversal plan. Each herb offers unique therapeutic benefits and can be tailored to meet the individual needs and preferences of individuals with diabetes seeking to improve their metabolic health and achieve sustainable reversal of the disease. As with any herbal treatment plan, it's important to consult with a qualified healthcare provider, such as Dr. Barbara, to ensure safety, efficacy, and compatibility with existing medical conditions or medications.

CHAPTER SEVEN

Nutritional Recommendations for Managing Diabetes

Diet plays a crucial role in the management of diabetes, influencing blood sugar control, insulin sensitivity, weight management, and overall health outcomes. Dr. Barbara's nutritional recommendations for managing diabetes focus on adopting a balanced, nutrient-rich diet that supports optimal metabolic function, stabilizes blood sugar levels, and reduces the risk of diabetes-related complications. These recommendations are tailored to individual needs, preferences, and health goals, aiming to empower individuals with diabetes to make informed dietary choices and achieve long-term success in managing their condition.

1. Emphasize Whole, Unprocessed Foods:

- Prioritize whole, unprocessed foods such as fruits, vegetables, whole grains, legumes, nuts, seeds, and lean proteins.

- These foods are rich in fiber, vitamins, minerals, and antioxidants, which support overall health and help stabilize blood sugar levels by slowing down the absorption of glucose into the bloodstream.

2. Focus on Low-Glycemic Index (GI) Foods:

- Choose carbohydrate-containing foods with a low glycemic index (GI) to minimize fluctuations in blood sugar levels.

- Low-GI foods include non-starchy vegetables, whole grains, legumes, nuts, seeds, and some fruits such as berries and citrus fruits.

3. Monitor Carbohydrate Intake:

- Pay attention to carbohydrate intake and distribute carbohydrates evenly throughout the day to prevent spikes and crashes in blood sugar levels.

- Aim for balanced meals that include a mix of carbohydrates, protein, and healthy fats to promote satiety and stabilize blood sugar levels.

4. Limit Added Sugars and Refined Carbohydrates:

- Minimize consumption of foods and beverages high in added sugars, refined grains, and processed carbohydrates, as these can lead to rapid increases in blood sugar levels.

- Choose whole, minimally processed sources of carbohydrates such as whole grains, fruits, and vegetables over sugary snacks, sweets, and sugary drinks.

5. Choose Healthy Fats:

- Include sources of healthy fats in your diet, such as avocados, nuts, seeds, olive oil, fatty fish (e.g., salmon, mackerel, sardines), and coconut oil.

- Healthy fats provide essential fatty acids, support heart health, and help regulate blood sugar levels by slowing down digestion and promoting satiety.

6. Prioritize Lean Proteins:

- Incorporate lean sources of protein into your meals and snacks, such as poultry, fish, tofu, tempeh, legumes, and low-fat dairy products.

- Protein-rich foods help stabilize blood sugar levels, promote muscle growth and repair, and contribute to feelings of fullness and satisfaction.

7. Portion Control and Mindful Eating:

- Practice portion control and mindful eating to avoid overeating and promote better blood sugar control.

- Pay attention to hunger and satiety cues, eat slowly, and savor each bite to enhance enjoyment and satisfaction from meals.

8. Stay Hydrated:

- Drink plenty of water throughout the day to stay hydrated and support optimal metabolic function.

- Limit consumption of sugary beverages, alcohol, and caffeinated drinks, which can contribute to dehydration and affect blood sugar levels.

9. Meal Planning and Preparation:

- Plan and prepare meals in advance to ensure consistency and adherence to dietary recommendations.

- Consider working with a registered dietitian or nutritionist to develop personalized meal plans and strategies for managing diabetes through nutrition.

10. Monitor Blood Sugar Levels:

- Regularly monitor blood sugar levels and track food intake, physical activity, and other relevant factors to identify patterns and make informed adjustments to your diet and lifestyle.

- Consult with a healthcare provider or diabetes educator for guidance on optimal blood sugar targets and monitoring frequency.

By incorporating these nutritional recommendations into your daily routine, you can effectively manage diabetes, improve metabolic health, and reduce the risk of complications associated with the condition. It's important to work closely with healthcare providers, such as Dr. Barbara, and a registered dietitian or nutritionist to develop a personalized nutrition plan tailored to your individual needs, preferences, and health goals. With commitment, education, and support, you can take control of your diabetes and lead a fulfilling, healthy life.

CHAPTER EIGHT

Lifestyle Modifications to Support Diabetes Reversal

In addition to dietary changes, lifestyle modifications play a crucial role in supporting diabetes reversal and improving overall metabolic health. Dr. Barbara emphasizes the importance of adopting healthy lifestyle habits that promote physical activity, stress management, adequate sleep, and overall well-being. These lifestyle modifications are tailored to individual needs and preferences, aiming to address underlying factors contributing to diabetes and facilitate sustainable long-term health outcomes. Here are key lifestyle modifications recommended by Dr. Barbara to support diabetes reversal:

1. Regular Physical Activity:

- Engage in regular aerobic exercise, strength training, and flexibility exercises to improve insulin sensitivity, regulate blood sugar levels, and promote weight management.

- Aim for at least 150 minutes of moderate-intensity aerobic activity or 75 minutes of vigorous-intensity aerobic activity per week, along with muscle-strengthening activities on two or more days per week.

2. Weight Management:

- Achieve and maintain a healthy weight through a combination of balanced nutrition, regular physical activity, and lifestyle modifications.

- Aim for gradual, sustainable weight loss if overweight or obese, as even modest weight reduction can lead to significant improvements in insulin sensitivity and metabolic health.

3. Stress Management:

- Practice stress-reducing techniques such as deep breathing exercises, meditation, mindfulness, yoga, tai chi, or progressive muscle relaxation to lower stress hormones and promote relaxation.

- Prioritize self-care activities, hobbies, and leisure pursuits that bring joy, fulfillment, and a sense of peace to your life.

4. Adequate Sleep:

- Prioritize getting sufficient sleep each night, aiming for 7-9 hours of restorative sleep for optimal metabolic health.

- Maintain a consistent sleep schedule, create a relaxing bedtime routine, and create a conducive sleep environment free of distractions, noise, and electronic devices.

5. Smoking Cessation:

- Quit smoking and avoid exposure to tobacco smoke, as smoking is associated with increased insulin resistance, higher risk of cardiovascular disease, and poorer diabetes outcomes.

- Seek support from healthcare providers, smoking cessation programs, or support groups to successfully quit smoking and improve overall health.

6. Limit Alcohol Consumption:

- Drink alcohol in moderation, if at all, as excessive alcohol consumption can interfere with blood sugar control, increase the risk of hypoglycemia, and contribute to weight gain.

- Follow guidelines for moderate alcohol consumption, which typically recommend up to one drink per day for women and up to two drinks per day for men.

7. Regular Monitoring and Follow-Up:

- Monitor blood sugar levels regularly as directed by healthcare providers and adjust treatment plans based on results.

- Attend regular follow-up appointments with healthcare providers, diabetes educators, and other members of the healthcare team to track progress, address concerns, and make necessary adjustments to the treatment plan.

8. Social Support and Community Engagement:

- Seek support from family members, friends, support groups, or online communities to share experiences, receive encouragement, and stay motivated on your diabetes reversal journey.

- Engage in social activities, volunteer work, or community events to foster connections, reduce isolation, and promote emotional well-being.

9. Education and Self-Management:

- Educate yourself about diabetes, its management, and the importance of lifestyle modifications in achieving optimal health outcomes.

- Take an active role in self-management by monitoring blood sugar levels, adhering to medication regimens, following dietary recommendations, and incorporating regular physical activity into your daily routine.

10. Goal Setting and Accountability:

- Set realistic goals for diabetes reversal, weight management, physical activity, and other lifestyle modifications, and track progress over time.

- Hold yourself accountable for meeting your goals, seek support from healthcare providers or health coaches, and celebrate achievements along the way.

By implementing these lifestyle modifications, individuals with diabetes can support the reversal of the condition, improve metabolic health, and reduce the risk of diabetes-related complications. Dr. Barbara emphasizes the importance of personalized lifestyle interventions tailored to individual needs and preferences, with guidance and support from healthcare providers, diabetes educators, and other members of the healthcare team. With commitment, consistency, and a holistic approach to wellness, individuals can achieve sustainable improvements in their health and well-being.

CHAPTER NINE

Monitoring Progress and Adjusting the Treatment Plan

Monitoring progress and making adjustments to the treatment plan are essential components of effective diabetes management and reversal. Dr. Barbara emphasizes the importance of regular assessment, monitoring, and personalized adjustments to ensure optimal outcomes and support individuals on their journey toward improved metabolic health. Here's a guide to monitoring progress and adjusting the treatment plan for individuals undergoing diabetes reversal:

1. Regular Health Check-ups:

- Schedule regular health check-ups with healthcare providers, including primary care physicians, endocrinologists, and diabetes educators.

- Monitor key indicators of metabolic health, such as blood sugar levels (fasting glucose, postprandial glucose, HbA1c), blood pressure, cholesterol levels, weight, and waist circumference.

2. Blood Glucose Monitoring:

- Monitor blood glucose levels regularly using self-monitoring devices, continuous glucose monitors (CGMs), or periodic laboratory tests as recommended by healthcare providers.

- Track patterns in blood sugar levels throughout the day, including fasting, pre-meal, postprandial, and bedtime readings, to identify trends and make informed adjustments to treatment.

3. Dietary Assessment:

- Conduct periodic dietary assessments to evaluate adherence to nutritional recommendations, identify areas for improvement, and make adjustments to the meal plan as needed.

- Review food logs, portion sizes, macronutrient distribution, and meal timing to ensure consistency and alignment with diabetes management goals.

4. Physical Activity Tracking:

- Monitor physical activity levels and exercise habits using activity trackers, exercise logs, or fitness apps to track frequency, duration, and intensity of exercise.

- Adjust exercise routines, intensity levels, and types of physical activity based on individual preferences, fitness level, and metabolic goals.

5. Medication Review:

- Review current medication regimens, including oral antidiabetic medications, insulin therapy, or other adjunctive therapies, to assess effectiveness, tolerability, and adherence.

- Consult with healthcare providers to make adjustments to medication dosages, schedules, or formulations based on changes in blood sugar levels, lifestyle factors, or treatment goals.

6. Lifestyle Assessment:

- Assess lifestyle factors, including stress levels, sleep quality, smoking habits, alcohol consumption, and social support networks, to identify areas for modification and support holistic well-being.

- Address underlying stressors, implement stress management techniques, and promote healthy coping strategies to reduce stress-related impacts on metabolic health.

7. Self-Monitoring and Goal Setting:

- Encourage individuals to engage in self-monitoring activities, such as keeping food journals, tracking physical activity, monitoring blood sugar levels, and recording lifestyle behaviors.

- Set realistic, achievable goals for diabetes management and reversal, and regularly review progress, celebrate achievements, and adjust goals as needed based on individual responses and outcomes.

8. Collaborative Care and Communication:

- Foster open communication and collaboration between individuals with diabetes and their healthcare providers, diabetes educators, nutritionists, and other members of the healthcare team.

- Encourage individuals to share concerns, ask questions, and actively participate in decision-making processes regarding treatment adjustments and lifestyle modifications.

9. Periodic Reassessment and Review:

- Schedule periodic reassessments and reviews of the treatment plan to evaluate progress, identify barriers or challenges, and make proactive adjustments to optimize outcomes.

- Incorporate feedback from individuals with diabetes regarding their experiences, preferences, and goals into the treatment planning process to ensure personalized, patient-centered care.

10. Ongoing Education and Support:

- Provide ongoing education, resources, and support to empower individuals with diabetes to make informed decisions, self-manage their condition, and maintain long-term adherence to lifestyle modifications.

- Offer access to support groups, educational workshops, online forums, and other community resources to enhance social support, peer interaction, and accountability.

By implementing a systematic approach to monitoring progress and adjusting the treatment plan, individuals with diabetes can optimize their outcomes, achieve sustainable improvements in metabolic health, and work toward the reversal of the condition. Dr. Barbara emphasizes the importance of personalized, patient-centered care that takes into account individual needs, preferences, and responses to treatment. With collaborative care, regular assessment, and proactive adjustments, individuals can take control of their diabetes management journey and achieve better health and well-being.

CHAPTER TEN

Success Stories and Testimonials: Experiences of Patients Reversing Diabetes with Dr. Barbara's Herbal Methods

Dr. Barbara's herbal methods for reversing diabetes have garnered numerous success stories and testimonials from individuals who have experienced significant improvements in their health and well-being. These testimonials highlight the transformative effects of Dr. Barbara's holistic approach to diabetes management, incorporating herbal remedies, dietary modifications, lifestyle interventions, and personalized care. Here are a few inspiring success stories from patients who have reversed diabetes with Dr. Barbara's guidance:

1. John's Journey to Diabetes Reversal:

- John, a 55-year-old man with type 2 diabetes, struggled for years to manage his blood sugar levels despite taking multiple medications and following conventional medical advice.

- After consulting with Dr. Barbara and adopting her herbal treatment protocol, John experienced remarkable improvements in his health within a few months.

- Through a combination of herbal supplements, dietary changes, and lifestyle modifications, John was able to achieve better blood sugar control, reduce his reliance on medications, and improve his overall quality of life.

- John's success story serves as an inspiration to others struggling with diabetes, demonstrating the effectiveness of Dr. Barbara's holistic approach in reversing the condition and restoring health.

2. Sarah's Transformation with Herbal Remedies:

- Sarah, a 45-year-old woman diagnosed with prediabetes, was determined to avoid progressing to full-blown diabetes and regain control of her health.

- With Dr. Barbara's guidance, Sarah embarked on a comprehensive herbal treatment plan that included targeted herbal supplements, dietary adjustments, and regular physical activity.

- Over the course of several months, Sarah saw dramatic improvements in her blood sugar levels, energy levels, and overall well-being.

- Through her dedication to Dr. Barbara's herbal methods and commitment to healthy lifestyle habits, Sarah successfully reversed prediabetes and restored her metabolic health, inspiring others to take charge of their health proactively.

3. James' Experience with Natural Healing:

- James, a 60-year-old man living with type 2 diabetes for over a decade, was frustrated with the limitations of conventional treatments and the side effects of medications.

- Seeking an alternative approach, James consulted with Dr. Barbara, who introduced him to the power of herbal medicine and holistic healing.

- With Dr. Barbara's guidance, James began incorporating herbal remedies, dietary changes, and stress management techniques into his daily routine.

- Over time, James experienced significant improvements in his blood sugar control, weight management, and overall health, allowing him to reduce his reliance on medications and regain a sense of vitality and well-being.

- James' journey exemplifies the transformative potential of Dr. Barbara's herbal methods in reversing diabetes and empowering individuals to reclaim their health naturally.

4. Maria's Success Story with Personalized Care:

- Maria, a 50-year-old woman diagnosed with gestational diabetes during her pregnancy, was determined to avoid developing type 2 diabetes later in life.

- With Dr. Barbara's personalized approach to care, Maria received tailored herbal remedies, dietary guidance, and lifestyle recommendations to address her unique health needs.

- Through consistent adherence to Dr. Barbara's treatment plan and ongoing support, Maria was able to successfully manage her blood sugar levels and prevent the onset of type 2 diabetes.

- Maria's journey highlights the importance of personalized care and holistic interventions in achieving optimal health outcomes and preventing chronic disease.

These success stories and testimonials are just a few examples of the transformative impact of Dr. Barbara's herbal methods in reversing diabetes and improving overall health and well-being. Each story underscores the effectiveness of Dr. Barbara's holistic approach, personalized care, and commitment to empowering individuals to take control of their health naturally. As more individuals share their experiences and achievements, Dr. Barbara's herbal methods continue to inspire hope and transformation in the lives of those affected by diabetes.

BONUS: SOME HOLISTIC AND HERBAL REMDIES YOU SHOULD KNOW

Bio Ferro Tonic:

Definition: Bio Ferro Tonic is a dietary supplement primarily composed of herbs and minerals. It's often marketed as a natural way to support overall health, particularly by promoting blood health and circulation.

Ingredients: Typical ingredients in Bio Ferro Tonic may include a blend of herbs such as burdock root, yellow dock root, sarsaparilla root, and cascara sagrada bark, along with minerals like iron and potassium phosphate.

How to Prepare: Bio Ferro Tonic usually comes in liquid form and is typically taken orally. It's important to follow the instructions on the product label for dosage and administration.

Dosage: The dosage can vary depending on the specific product and individual needs. It's crucial to consult with a healthcare professional or follow the recommended dosage on the product label to avoid potential side effects.

How to Use: Bio Ferro Tonic is often taken by adding the recommended dosage to water or juice and consuming it orally. It's important to shake the bottle well before use and store it according to the manufacturer's instructions.

Side Effects: While Bio Ferro Tonic is generally considered safe when used as directed, some individuals may experience side effects such as digestive discomfort, allergic reactions, or interactions with medications. It's essential to consult with a healthcare provider before starting any new supplement regimen, especially if you have underlying health conditions or are taking medications.

Bladderwrack:

Definition: Bladderwrack is a type of seaweed or marine algae commonly used in traditional medicine and as a dietary supplement. It's known for its potential health benefits, particularly related to thyroid health and weight management.

Ingredients: Bladderwrack contains various nutrients, including iodine, vitamins, minerals, and antioxidants. The primary active components are iodine and fucoidan, a type of carbohydrate found in brown seaweeds.

How to Prepare: Bladderwrack supplements are available in various forms, including capsules, powders, and liquid extracts. They can be taken orally with water or added to smoothies and other beverages.

Dosage: The appropriate dosage of bladderwrack can vary based on factors such as age, health status, and the specific product being used. It's essential to follow the recommended dosage on the product label or consult with a healthcare professional for personalized guidance.

How to Use: Bladderwrack supplements are typically taken orally, either with water or mixed into food or beverages. It's important to follow the instructions on the product label and avoid exceeding the recommended dosage.

Side Effects: While bladderwrack is generally considered safe for most people when used in moderation, excessive intake of iodine from bladderwrack supplements can cause thyroid dysfunction and other adverse effects. Individuals with thyroid disorders, iodine sensitivity, or certain medical conditions should exercise caution and consult with a healthcare provider before using bladderwrack supplements. Common side effects may include digestive upset, allergic reactions, or interactions with medications.

Blood Purifier:

Definition: Blood purifiers are herbal remedies or dietary supplements believed to cleanse or detoxify the blood, often promoting overall health and well-being. They are thought to support the body's natural detoxification processes and improve blood circulation.

Ingredients: Blood purifiers may contain a variety of herbs and botanical extracts known for their purported cleansing and detoxifying properties. Common ingredients include burdock root, red clover, dandelion root, and yellow dock root, among others.

How to Prepare: Blood purifiers are typically available in various forms, including capsules, tablets, powders, and liquid extracts. They are usually taken orally with water or juice, following the recommended dosage on the product label.

Dosage: The dosage of blood purifiers can vary depending on the specific product and individual needs. It's important to adhere to the recommended dosage on the product label or consult with a healthcare professional for personalized guidance.

How to Use: Blood purifiers are typically taken orally, either with water or mixed into beverages. They are often used as part of a detoxification regimen or to support overall health and vitality.

Side Effects: While blood purifiers are generally considered safe for most people when used as directed, some individuals may experience side effects such as digestive discomfort, allergic reactions, or interactions with medications. It's important to consult with a healthcare provider before starting any new supplement regimen, especially if you have underlying health conditions or are taking medications.

Burdock:

Definition: Burdock, scientifically known as Arctium lappa, is a biennial plant native to Europe and Asia but now found worldwide. It's part of the Asteraceae family and has been used for centuries in traditional medicine and culinary practices.

Ingredients: Burdock contains various nutrients, including carbohydrates, fiber, vitamins (such as vitamin B6, folate, and vitamin C), and minerals (including potassium, magnesium, and manganese). It also contains active compounds such as polyphenols and volatile oils.

How to Prepare: Burdock can be prepared and consumed in various ways. The roots, leaves, and seeds are all utilized for different purposes. The root is commonly used in cooking, herbal teas, tinctures, and supplements, while the leaves and seeds are sometimes used in herbal preparations.

Dosage: The appropriate dosage of burdock root can vary depending on the specific form and intended use. For culinary purposes, there are no strict dosage guidelines, but for supplements or herbal remedies, it's essential to follow the recommended dosage on the product label or consult with a healthcare professional.

How to Use: Burdock root can be used in cooking by peeling, slicing, and adding it to soups, stews, stir-fries, or salads. It can also be brewed into a tea or used to make tinctures or extracts for medicinal purposes. Some people may also take burdock root supplements in capsule or powder form.

Side Effects: While burdock is generally considered safe for most people when consumed in moderate amounts, some individuals may experience allergic reactions or digestive upset. Additionally, burdock may interact with certain medications or have adverse effects in individuals with certain health conditions, such as diabetes or allergies to plants in the Asteraceae family. It's important to consult with a healthcare provider before using burdock, especially if you have underlying health conditions or are taking medications.

Cascara Sagrada:

Definition: Cascara Sagrada, scientifically known as Rhamnus purshiana, is a species of buckthorn native to western North America. It has been used traditionally as a laxative and to promote bowel regularity.

Ingredients: The primary active ingredients in cascara sagrada are anthraquinone glycosides, particularly cascarosides A and B. These compounds stimulate peristalsis in the colon, leading to increased bowel movements.

How to Prepare: Cascara sagrada is typically prepared as an herbal tea, tincture, or capsule. To make tea, dried cascara sagrada bark is steeped in hot water for several minutes before being strained and consumed. Tinctures are prepared by steeping the bark in alcohol to extract its active compounds.

Dosage: The appropriate dosage of cascara sagrada can vary depending on the specific preparation and intended use. It's important to follow the recommended dosage on the product label or consult with a healthcare professional for personalized guidance.

How to Use: Cascara sagrada tea or tincture is typically taken orally. It's important to start with a low dose and gradually increase if needed to avoid potential side effects such as cramping or diarrhea.

Side Effects: Cascara sagrada is considered safe for short-term use when used as directed. However, long-term or excessive use may lead to dependence, electrolyte imbalance, or dehydration. It may also interact with certain medications or have adverse effects in individuals with certain health conditions. It's important to use cascara sagrada under the guidance of a healthcare professional and to discontinue use if any adverse effects occur.

Cell Food:

Definition: Cell Food is a dietary supplement marketed as a highly oxygenating and alkalizing formula. It's claimed to support overall health and vitality by providing essential nutrients and oxygen to the cells.

Ingredients: The exact ingredients of Cell Food can vary depending on the brand, but it typically contains a proprietary blend of minerals, enzymes, electrolytes, and trace elements. Some common ingredients may include purified water, dissolved oxygen, seawater extract, and plant-based enzymes.

How to Prepare: Cell Food is usually available in liquid form and is typically taken orally. It can be consumed directly or diluted in water or juice before consumption.

Dosage: The dosage of Cell Food can vary depending on the specific product and individual needs. It's important to follow the recommended dosage on the product label or consult with a healthcare professional for personalized guidance.

How to Use: Cell Food is typically taken orally, either directly or mixed into water or juice. It's important to shake the bottle well before use and to store it according to the manufacturer's instructions.

Side Effects: Cell Food is generally considered safe for most people when used as directed. However, some individuals may experience mild digestive upset or allergic reactions to certain ingredients. It's essential to consult with a healthcare provider before starting any new supplement regimen, especially if you have underlying health conditions or are taking medications.

Chaparral:

Definition: Chaparral, scientifically known as Larrea tridentata, is a shrub native to the southwestern United States and northern Mexico. It has been used for centuries by Native American tribes for its medicinal properties and is commonly used in herbal medicine today.

Ingredients: Chaparral contains several bioactive compounds, including nordihydroguaiaretic acid (NDGA), flavonoids, lignans, and volatile oils. NDGA is believed to be the primary active compound responsible for many of chaparral's therapeutic effects.

How to Prepare: Chaparral can be prepared and consumed in various forms, including teas, tinctures, capsules, and topical preparations. To make tea, dried chaparral leaves are steeped in hot water for several minutes before being strained and consumed. Tinctures are prepared by steeping the herb in alcohol or vinegar to extract its active compounds.

Dosage: The appropriate dosage of chaparral can vary depending on the specific form and intended use. It's important to follow the recommended dosage on the product label or consult with a healthcare professional for personalized guidance.

How to Use: Chaparral tea or tincture is typically taken orally. It can also be applied topically to the skin for certain conditions. It's important to use chaparral products as directed and to discontinue use if any adverse effects occur.

Side Effects: Chaparral is generally considered safe for most people when used in moderate amounts. However, excessive intake or prolonged use may lead to liver toxicity or other adverse effects. It may also interact with certain medications or have adverse effects in individuals with certain health conditions. It's important to use chaparral under the guidance of a healthcare professional and to discontinue use if any adverse effects occur.

Cocolmeca:

Definition: Cocolmeca, also known as Smilax ornata or sarsaparilla, is a flowering vine native to Mexico and Central America. It has been used traditionally in Mexican and Central American folk medicine for its purported medicinal properties.

Ingredients: Cocolmeca contains various bioactive compounds, including saponins, flavonoids, and plant sterols. These compounds are believed to contribute to the herb's medicinal properties, including its potential as a diuretic, blood purifier, and anti-inflammatory agent.

How to Prepare: Cocolmeca is commonly prepared and consumed as an herbal tea or decoction. To make tea, dried cocolmeca roots or leaves are steeped in hot water for several minutes before being strained and consumed. Decoctions involve boiling the roots or leaves in water to extract their active compounds.

Dosage: The appropriate dosage of cocolmeca can vary depending on factors such as age, health status, and the specific preparation being used. It's important to follow the recommended dosage on the product label or consult with a qualified herbalist or healthcare professional for personalized guidance.

How to Use: Cocolmeca tea or decoction is typically taken orally. It can also be used topically for certain skin conditions. It's important to use cocolmeca products as directed and to discontinue use if any adverse effects occur.

Side Effects: Cocolmeca is generally considered safe for most people when used in moderate amounts. However, excessive intake may lead to digestive upset or other adverse effects. It may also interact with certain medications or have adverse effects in individuals with certain health conditions. It's important to use cocolmeca under the guidance of a healthcare professional and to discontinue use if any adverse effects occur.

Contribo:

Definition: Contribo, also known as Aristolochiatrilobata, is a vine native to the Caribbean and Central America. It has been used traditionally in folk medicine for various purposes, including as a remedy for digestive issues, inflammation, and pain relief.

Ingredients: Contribo contains several bioactive compounds, including aristolochic acids, flavonoids, and alkaloids. These compounds are believed to contribute to the herb's medicinal properties, including its potential as an anti-inflammatory and analgesic agent.

How to Prepare: Contribo is typically prepared and consumed as an herbal tea or decoction. To make tea, dried contribo leaves or stems are steeped in hot water for several minutes before being strained and consumed. Decoctions involve boiling the leaves or stems in water to extract their active compounds.

Dosage: The appropriate dosage of contribo can vary depending on factors such as age, health status, and the specific preparation being used. It's important to follow the recommended dosage on the product label or consult with a qualified herbalist or healthcare professional for personalized guidance.

How to Use: Contribo tea or decoction is typically taken orally. It's important to use contribo products as directed and to discontinue use if any adverse effects occur.

Side Effects: Contribo contains aristolochic acids, which have been associated with serious adverse effects, including kidney damage and cancer. Due to these safety concerns, the use of contribo is highly discouraged, and it's important to avoid products containing aristolochic acids. Individuals should seek alternative remedies for their health needs.

Dandelion Root:

Definition: Dandelion, scientifically known as Taraxacum officinale, is a common flowering plant found worldwide. While often considered a pesky weed, dandelion has a long history of use in traditional medicine for its various health benefits.

Ingredients: Dandelion root contains several bioactive compounds, including sesquiterpene lactones, triterpenes, flavonoids, and polysaccharides. These compounds are believed to contribute to the herb's medicinal properties, including its potential as a diuretic, digestive aid, and liver tonic.

How to Prepare: Dandelion root can be prepared and consumed in various forms, including teas, tinctures, capsules, and extracts. To make tea, dried dandelion root is steeped in hot water for several minutes before being strained and consumed. Tinctures are prepared by steeping the root in alcohol or vinegar to extract its active compounds.

Dosage: The appropriate dosage of dandelion root can vary depending on factors such as age, health status, and the specific preparation being used. It's important to follow the recommended dosage on the product label or consult with a qualified herbalist or healthcare professional for personalized guidance.

How to Use: Dandelion root tea, tincture, or capsules are typically taken orally. It's important to use dandelion root products as directed and to discontinue use if any adverse effects occur.

Side Effects: Dandelion root is generally considered safe for most people when used in moderate amounts. However, some individuals may experience allergic reactions or digestive upset. It may also interact with certain medications or have adverse effects in individuals with certain health conditions. It's important to use dandelion root under the guidance of a healthcare professional and to discontinue use if any adverse effects occur.

Green Food Plus:

Definition: Green Food Plus is a dietary supplement formulated to provide a concentrated source of nutrients derived from various green plants. It's designed to support overall health and well-being by delivering essential vitamins, minerals, antioxidants, and phytonutrients.

Ingredients: Green Food Plus typically contains a blend of powdered green vegetables, grasses, algae, and other plant-based ingredients. Common ingredients may include wheatgrass, barley grass, spirulina, chlorella, alfalfa, kale, spinach, and broccoli, among others.

How to Prepare: Green Food Plus is usually available in powder form and can be mixed with water, juice, or smoothies. It's important to follow the recommended dosage on the product label and to consume it as part of a balanced diet.

Dosage: The appropriate dosage of Green Food Plus can vary depending on the specific product and individual needs. It's important to follow the recommended dosage on the product label or consult with a healthcare professional for personalized guidance.

How to Use: Green Food Plus powder is typically mixed with water, juice, or smoothies and consumed orally. It's often taken once or twice daily, preferably with meals, to maximize nutrient absorption.

Side Effects: Green Food Plus is generally considered safe for most people when used as directed. However, some individuals may experience digestive upset or allergic reactions to certain ingredients. It's important to consult with a healthcare provider before starting any new supplement regimen, especially if you have underlying health conditions or are taking medications.

Hydrangea:

Definition: Hydrangea, scientifically known as Hydrangea arborescens, is a flowering shrub native to North America. It has been used traditionally in herbal medicine for its potential diuretic and anti-inflammatory properties.

Ingredients: Hydrangea contains several bioactive compounds, including saponins, flavonoids, and glycosides. These compounds are believed to contribute to the herb's medicinal properties, including its potential as a diuretic, kidney tonic, and anti-inflammatory agent.

How to Prepare: Hydrangea root is typically prepared and consumed as an herbal tea or tincture. To make tea, dried hydrangea root is steeped in hot water for several minutes before being strained and consumed. Tinctures are prepared by steeping the root in alcohol or vinegar to extract its active compounds.

Dosage: The appropriate dosage of hydrangea can vary depending on factors such as age, health status, and the specific preparation being used. It's important to follow the recommended dosage on the product label or consult with a qualified herbalist or healthcare professional for personalized guidance.

How to Use: Hydrangea tea or tincture is typically taken orally. It's important to use hydrangea products as directed and to discontinue use if any adverse effects occur.

Side Effects: Hydrangea is generally considered safe for most people when used in moderate amounts. However, some individuals may experience digestive upset or allergic reactions. It may also interact with certain medications or have adverse effects in individuals with certain health conditions. It's important to use hydrangea under the guidance of a healthcare professional and to discontinue use if any adverse effects occur.

Irish Moss:

Definition: Irish Moss, scientifically known as Chondrus crispus, is a species of red algae or seaweed native to the Atlantic coastlines of Europe and North America. It has been used for centuries in traditional Irish and Scottish cuisine, as well as in herbal medicine.

Ingredients: Irish Moss is rich in various nutrients, including iodine, sulfur compounds, vitamins (such as vitamin A, vitamin K, and vitamin B12), minerals (including calcium, magnesium, potassium, and sodium), and polysaccharides (such as carrageenan). These nutrients are believed to contribute to the herb's potential health benefits.

How to Prepare: Irish Moss is typically prepared by soaking it in water to rehydrate and soften it before use. It can be added to soups, stews, smoothies, desserts, and other dishes as a thickening agent or nutritional supplement.

Dosage: The appropriate dosage of Irish Moss can vary depending on factors such as age, health status, and the specific preparation being used. It's important to follow recipes or guidelines for culinary use and to consult with a healthcare professional for guidance on using Irish Moss as a dietary supplement.

How to Use: Irish Moss can be used in culinary applications to add thickness and nutritional value to dishes. It can also be consumed as a dietary supplement in the form of capsules, powders, or extracts.

Side Effects: Irish Moss is generally considered safe for most people when consumed in moderate amounts as part of a balanced diet. However, some individuals may be allergic to seaweed or carrageenan, a compound found in Irish Moss that is used as a food additive. It's important to discontinue use if any adverse effects occur and to consult with a healthcare professional if you have any concerns.

Irish Sea Moss:

Definition: Irish Sea Moss is a term often used interchangeably with Irish Moss, referring to the same species of red algae, Chondrus crispus. It's harvested from the rocky shores of the Atlantic coastlines of Europe and North America.

Ingredients: Irish Sea Moss shares the same nutritional profile as Irish Moss, containing iodine, vitamins, minerals, and polysaccharides. It's valued for its potential health benefits, including supporting thyroid function, boosting immune health, and promoting digestion.

How to Prepare: Irish Sea Moss is prepared in the same way as Irish Moss, by soaking it in water to rehydrate and soften it before use. It can be used in culinary applications or consumed as a dietary supplement.

Dosage: The dosage of Irish Sea Moss depends on the form and intended use. As a dietary supplement, it's important to follow the recommended dosage on the product label or consult with a healthcare professional for personalized guidance.

How to Use: Irish Sea Moss can be used in various culinary applications, including soups, smoothies, desserts, and sauces. It can also be consumed as a dietary supplement in the form of capsules, powders, or extracts.

Side Effects: Similar to Irish Moss, Irish Sea Moss is generally considered safe for most people when consumed in moderate amounts. However, individuals with seaweed allergies or sensitivities to carrageenan should exercise caution. It's important to discontinue use if any adverse effects occur and to consult with a healthcare professional if you have any concerns.

Red Clover:

Definition: Red clover, scientifically known as Trifolium pratense, is a flowering plant belonging to the legume family. It's native to Europe, Western Asia, and Northwest Africa but has been naturalized in many other regions. Red clover has been used in traditional medicine for various purposes, including its potential to support women's health and menopausal symptoms.

Ingredients: Red clover contains several bioactive compounds, including isoflavones (such as genistein and daidzein), flavonoids, and phytoestrogens. These compounds are believed to contribute to the herb's medicinal properties, including its potential as a hormone-balancing agent and its ability to support cardiovascular health.

How to Prepare: Red clover is typically prepared and consumed as an herbal tea or tincture. To make tea, dried red clover flowers are steeped in hot water for several minutes before being strained and consumed. Tinctures are prepared by steeping the flowers in alcohol or vinegar to extract their active compounds.

Dosage: The appropriate dosage of red clover can vary depending on factors such as age, health status, and the specific preparation being used. It's important to follow the recommended dosage on the product label or consult with a qualified herbalist or healthcare professional for personalized guidance.

How to Use: Red clover tea or tincture is typically taken orally. It's important to use red clover products as directed and to discontinue use if any adverse effects occur.

Side Effects: Red clover is generally considered safe for most people when used in moderate amounts. However, some individuals may experience allergic reactions or digestive upset. It may also interact with certain medications or have adverse effects in individuals with certain health conditions. It's important to use red clover under the guidance of a healthcare professional and to discontinue use if any adverse effects occur.

Red Raspberry:

Definition: Red raspberry, scientifically known as Rubus idaeus, is a species of raspberry native to Europe and northern Asia. It's widely cultivated for its delicious berries and has been used in traditional medicine for various purposes, including its potential to support women's health during pregnancy and childbirth.

Ingredients: Red raspberry contains several bioactive compounds, including flavonoids, ellagic acid, anthocyanins, and vitamin C. These compounds are believed to contribute to the herb's medicinal properties, including its potential as an antioxidant, anti-inflammatory, and uterine tonic.

How to Prepare: Red raspberry leaf is typically prepared and consumed as an herbal tea or infusion. To make tea, dried red raspberry leaves are steeped in hot water for several minutes before being strained and consumed.

Dosage: The appropriate dosage of red raspberry leaf can vary depending on factors such as age, health status, and the specific preparation being used. It's important to follow the recommended dosage on the product label or consult with a qualified herbalist or healthcare professional for personalized guidance.

How to Use: Red raspberry leaf tea is typically taken orally. It's often recommended for pregnant individuals in the later stages of pregnancy to support uterine health and prepare for childbirth. It's important to use red raspberry leaf products as directed and to discontinue use if any adverse effects occur.

Side Effects: Red raspberry leaf is generally considered safe for most people when used in moderate amounts. However, some individuals may experience allergic reactions or digestive upset. Pregnant individuals should consult with a healthcare professional before using red raspberry leaf, especially if they have any underlying health conditions or are taking medications. It's important to use red raspberry leaf under the guidance of a healthcare professional and to discontinue use if any adverse effects occur.

Lymphalin:

Definition: Lymphalin is a herbal supplement formulated to support lymphatic system health. The lymphatic system plays a crucial role in immune function and waste removal in the body, and Lymphalin is designed to promote its proper function.

Ingredients: Lymphalin typically contains a blend of herbs and botanical extracts known for their traditional use in supporting lymphatic system health. Common ingredients may include cleavers, red clover, echinacea, burdock root, and calendula, among others.

How to Prepare: Lymphalin is usually available in capsule or liquid form. Capsules are taken orally with water, while liquid forms may be mixed with water or juice before consumption. It's important to follow the recommended dosage on the product label.

Dosage: The appropriate dosage of Lymphalin can vary depending on the specific product and individual needs. It's important to follow the recommended dosage on the product label or consult with a healthcare professional for personalized guidance.

How to Use: Lymphalin capsules are typically taken orally with water, while liquid forms may be mixed with water or juice before consumption. It's often recommended to take Lymphalin on an empty stomach for optimal absorption.

Side Effects: Lymphalin is generally considered safe for most people when used as directed. However, some individuals may experience mild side effects such as gastrointestinal discomfort or allergic reactions to certain ingredients. It's important to consult with a healthcare provider before starting any new supplement regimen, especially if you have underlying health conditions or are taking medications.

Manjakani:

Definition: Manjakani, also known as Quercus infectoria or oak gall, is a natural substance derived from the oak tree. It has been used for centuries in traditional medicine for its potential health benefits, particularly for women's health and vaginal tightening.

Ingredients: Manjakani contains various bioactive compounds, including tannins, flavonoids, and gallic acid. These compounds are believed to contribute to the herb's medicinal properties, including its potential as an astringent and antiseptic agent.

How to Prepare: Manjakani is typically available in powder, capsule, or liquid extract form. It can be taken orally or used topically depending on the intended use. For vaginal tightening, manjakani may be applied topically as a gel or inserted into the vagina in capsule form.

Dosage: The appropriate dosage of manjakani can vary depending on factors such as age, health status, and the specific preparation being used. It's important to follow the recommended dosage on the product label or consult with a qualified herbalist or healthcare professional for personalized guidance.

How to Use: Manjakani can be taken orally or used topically depending on the intended use. It's important to use manjakani products as directed and to discontinue use if any adverse effects occur.

Side Effects: Manjakani is generally considered safe for most people when used in moderate amounts. However, some individuals may experience allergic reactions or skin irritation when used topically. It's important to use manjakani under the guidance of a healthcare professional and to discontinue use if any adverse effects occur.

Guaco:

Definition: Guaco, also known as Mikania cordata or Mikania glomerata, is a medicinal plant native to Central and South America. It has a long history of use in traditional medicine for its potential therapeutic properties.

Ingredients: Guaco contains several bioactive compounds, including coumarins, flavonoids, tannins, and saponins. These compounds are believed to contribute to the herb's medicinal properties, including its potential as an expectorant, anti-inflammatory, and antispasmodic agent.

How to Prepare: Guaco is typically prepared and consumed as an herbal tea or infusion. To make tea, dried guaco leaves are steeped in hot water for several minutes before being strained and consumed.

Dosage: The appropriate dosage of guaco can vary depending on factors such as age, health status, and the specific preparation being used. It's important to follow the recommended dosage on the product label or consult with a qualified herbalist or healthcare professional for personalized guidance.

How to Use: Guaco tea is typically taken orally. It can be consumed on its own or mixed with honey or other herbal teas for added flavor.

Side Effects: Guaco is generally considered safe for most people when used in moderate amounts. However, some individuals may experience allergic reactions or digestive upset. It may also interact with certain medications or have adverse effects in individuals with certain health conditions. It's important to use guaco under the guidance of a healthcare professional and to discontinue use if any adverse effects occur.

Herban Iron:

Definition: Herban Iron is a dietary supplement designed to provide an easily absorbable form of iron to support healthy iron levels in the body. It's particularly beneficial for individuals with iron deficiency or anemia.

Ingredients: Herban Iron typically contains iron in the form of ferrous bisglycinate, which is a highly bioavailable and gentle form of iron that is less likely to cause digestive upset or constipation compared to other forms of iron. It may also contain other ingredients such as vitamin C to enhance iron absorption.

How to Prepare: Herban Iron is usually available in capsule or liquid form. Capsules are taken orally with water, while liquid forms may be mixed with water or juice before consumption. It's important to follow the recommended dosage on the product label.

Dosage: The appropriate dosage of Herban Iron depends on factors such as age, gender, and the severity of iron deficiency. It's important to consult with a healthcare professional to determine the correct dosage for individual needs.

How to Use: Herban Iron capsules are typically taken orally with water, while liquid forms may be mixed with water or juice before consumption. It's important to take Herban Iron as directed and to avoid taking it with dairy products, antacids, or other substances that may interfere with iron absorption.

Side Effects: While Herban Iron is generally considered safe for most people when used as directed, some individuals may experience mild side effects such as gastrointestinal discomfort or constipation. It's important to consult with a healthcare professional before starting any new supplement regimen, especially if you have underlying health conditions or are taking medications.

Blue Vervain:

Definition: Blue vervain, also known as Verbena hastata, is a perennial herb native to North America. It has been used in traditional medicine for centuries to treat various ailments, including anxiety, insomnia, and digestive issues.

Ingredients: Blue vervain contains several active compounds, including aucubin, verbenalin, and volatile oils. These compounds are believed to contribute to the herb's medicinal properties.

How to Prepare: Blue vervain is typically consumed as a tea or tincture. To make tea, dried blue vervain leaves and flowers are steeped in hot water for several minutes before being strained and consumed. Tinctures are prepared by steeping the herb in alcohol or vinegar to extract its active compounds.

Dosage: The appropriate dosage of blue vervain can vary depending on factors such as age, health status, and the specific preparation being used. It's important to follow the recommended dosage on the product label or consult with a qualified herbalist or healthcare professional for personalized guidance.

How to Use: Blue vervain tea or tincture is typically taken orally. It can be consumed on its own or mixed with honey or other herbal teas for added flavor.

Side Effects: While blue vervain is generally considered safe for most people when used in moderation, excessive intake may cause digestive upset or allergic reactions in some individuals. Pregnant or breastfeeding women should avoid blue vervain due to its potential to stimulate uterine contractions. As with any herbal remedy, it's important to consult with a healthcare provider before using blue vervain, especially if you have underlying health conditions or are taking medications.

Bromide Plus Powder:

Definition: Bromide Plus Powder is a dietary supplement formulated to support thyroid health and promote overall well-being. It typically contains a blend of herbs and minerals that are believed to have beneficial effects on thyroid function.

Ingredients: Bromide Plus Powder often contains a combination of herbs such as bladderwrack, sea moss, and burdock root, along with minerals like iodine and potassium phosphate. These ingredients are thought to support thyroid function and maintain optimal iodine levels in the body.

How to Prepare: Bromide Plus Powder is usually mixed with water or juice to create a drinkable solution. It's important to follow the instructions on the product label for dosage and preparation.

Dosage: The dosage of Bromide Plus Powder can vary depending on the specific product and individual needs. It's crucial to consult with a healthcare professional or follow the recommended dosage on the product label to avoid potential side effects.

How to Use: Bromide Plus Powder is typically taken orally by mixing the recommended dosage with water or juice. It's important to shake or stir the mixture well before consuming it to ensure even distribution of the ingredients.

Side Effects: While Bromide Plus Powder is generally considered safe when used as directed, some individuals may experience side effects such as digestive discomfort or allergic reactions to certain ingredients. It's essential to consult with a healthcare provider before starting any new supplement regimen, especially if you have underlying health conditions or are taking medications.

Bugleweed:

Definition: Bugleweed, also known as Lycopusvirginicus, is a perennial herb native to North America and Europe. It has been used in traditional medicine to treat various conditions, including hyperthyroidism, anxiety, and insomnia.

Ingredients: Bugleweed contains several active compounds, including lithospermic acid, phenolic acids, and flavonoids. These compounds are believed to contribute to the herb's medicinal properties, particularly its ability to regulate thyroid function.

How to Prepare: Bugleweed is commonly consumed as a tea or tincture. To make tea, dried bugleweed leaves and flowers are steeped in hot water for several minutes before being strained and consumed. Tinctures are prepared by steeping the herb in alcohol or vinegar to extract its active compounds.

Dosage: The appropriate dosage of bugleweed can vary depending on factors such as age, health status, and the specific preparation being used. It's important to follow the recommended dosage on the product label or consult with a qualified herbalist or healthcare professional for personalized guidance.

How to Use: Bugleweed tea or tincture is typically taken orally. It can be consumed on its own or mixed with honey or other herbal teas for added flavor.

Side Effects: While bugleweed is generally considered safe for most people when used in moderation, excessive intake may cause digestive upset or allergic reactions in some individuals. Pregnant or breastfeeding women should avoid bugleweed due to its potential to stimulate uterine contractions. As with any herbal remedy, it's important to consult with a healthcare provider before using bugleweed, especially if you have underlying health conditions or are taking medications.

THE END

www.ingramcontent.com/pod-product-compliance
Lightning Source LLC
Chambersburg PA
CBHW081558250726
48653CB00009B/3484

9 798327 233966